The Art of Pranayama

Mastering the Breath for Mind, Body, and Spirit a Power of Breath work to cultivate a Harmonious Life

Lewis Finan

Table of Contents

Introduction

In the hustle and bustle of modern life, where stress and distractions seem to be the norm, there exists a timeless practice that has the power to reconnect us with the essence of our being – the art of Pranayama. This ancient discipline, rooted in the rich traditions of yoga and breathwork, offers a profound journey towards mastering the breath for the betterment of our mind, body, and spirit.

"The Art of Pranayama: Mastering the Breath for Mind, Body, and Spirit" is a guide that invites you to explore the transformative potential of conscious breathing. Pranayama, derived from Sanskrit, translates to the control (yama) of life force (prana). It is not just a physical act of inhaling and exhaling but an exploration into the very essence of our vitality and consciousness.

As we navigate the challenges of the modern world, we often forget the simple yet profound act of breathing – an innate process that sustains our existence. The book delves into the principles and practices of Pranayama, illuminating the intricate connection between breath and our overall well-being. Through the power of breathwork, we can unlock the door to inner harmony and cultivate a life that resonates with balance and tranquility.

This comprehensive guide is designed for both beginners and seasoned practitioners, offering a step-by-step journey into the various techniques of Pranayama. From foundational practices to advanced breath control, each chapter unfolds a new dimension of understanding, guiding you towards mastery of the breath that extends beyond the yoga mat into every facet of your life.

Beyond the physical benefits of improved lung capacity and enhanced vitality, Pranayama serves as a gateway to self-discovery and spiritual awakening. It teaches us to be present in each breath, fostering mindfulness and awareness. The practices shared within these pages have the potential to alleviate stress, anxiety, and emotional turbulence, providing a pathway to a harmonious and balanced life.

Join us on this exploration of the art of Pranayama – a journey that transcends the boundaries of time and culture. As we tap into the power of breath, we discover a reservoir of energy and wisdom that can transform our lives. May this book be your companion in unlocking the secrets of breath, guiding you toward a life that resonates with the harmonious rhythm of existence.

Understanding Pranayama

Pranayama, a cornerstone of yogic philosophy, is an ancient practice that delves into the profound relationship between breath, energy, and consciousness. Derived from Sanskrit, where "prana" means life force or vital energy, and "Yama" implies control, Pranayama is the art of consciously regulating the breath to attain physical, mental, and spiritual well-being.

At its core, Pranayama recognizes that breath is more than a physiological process—it is a bridge between the body and the mind, a vehicle for the life force that animates us. The practice involves a deliberate and disciplined approach to breathing, acknowledging the transformative power inherent in the simple act of inhaling and exhaling.

The principles of Pranayama are deeply rooted in ancient texts such as the Yoga Sutras of Patanjali, which it is considered one of the eight limbs of yoga. Here, breath is seen as a medium to quiet the fluctuations of the mind and connect with a higher state of consciousness. Through various techniques, practitioners learn to harness and direct the flow of prana within the body, promoting physical health, mental clarity, and spiritual awareness.

One fundamental aspect of Pranayama is the awareness of breath patterns. The practice encourages individuals to observe the natural rhythm of their breathing and, through conscious effort, modify it to achieve specific effects. Techniques range from simple breath awareness (anulom vilom) to more intricate breath retention (kumbhaka), each serving a unique purpose in promoting balance and vitality.

Pranayama is not confined to the yoga studio; it is a practical tool that can be integrated into daily life. The breath becomes a guide, helping individuals navigate stress, emotions, and challenges with equanimity. Beyond the physical benefits of increased lung capacity and oxygenation, practitioners often report heightened states of relaxation, improved focus, and a greater sense of inner peace.

This exploration into the heart of Pranayama invites you to embark on a journey of self-discovery, tapping into the wisdom of ancient practices to cultivate a harmonious life. As we unravel the layers of breath, energy, and consciousness, may you find not only a deeper understanding of Pranayama but also a transformative path toward holistic well-being.

The Importance of Breath in Daily Life

In the tapestry of daily living, where demands and distractions abound, there exists a constant and often overlooked companion—the breath. Beyond its essential role in sustaining life, the breath holds a profound significance in shaping the quality of our existence. Understanding and harnessing the power of breath can be a transformative key to unlocking a myriad of physical, mental, and emotional benefits.

At its most fundamental level, breath is the rhythmic exchange of air that sustains the body's vital functions. Yet, its importance transcends mere oxygenation. The way we breathe has a direct impact on our physiological state, influencing heart rate, blood pressure, and stress levels. Shallow, rapid breathing can trigger the body's stress response, while slow, deliberate breaths have the potential to induce a state of calm and relaxation.

In the chaos of daily life, stress has become an unwelcome companion for many. The breath, however, emerges as a powerful antidote. Mindful and intentional breathing serves as a bridge between the autonomic nervous system's sympathetic (fight-or-flight) and parasympathetic (rest-and-digest) branches. By consciously regulating our breath, we can shift from a state of heightened alertness to a calmer, more centered presence.

Moreover, the breath is a mirror reflecting the state of the mind. When the mind is agitated, the breath often follows suit—quick and erratic. Conversely, a tranquil mind is mirrored in a steady and even breath. Recognizing this interconnection, various contemplative traditions and wellness practices emphasize the importance of cultivating a harmonious relationship between mind and breath.

Incorporating conscious breathing into daily life is accessible to everyone, irrespective of age or physical condition. Simple techniques, such as diaphragmatic breathing or focused breath awareness, can be seamlessly integrated into routine activities. Whether commuting, working, or facing moments of tension, a few moments of intentional breathing can act as a reset button, bringing clarity and a sense of balance.

Furthermore, the breath serves as a gateway to mindfulness—a practice gaining recognition for its ability to enhance overall well-being. By anchoring our attention to the present moment through the breath, we foster a heightened awareness that extends beyond the confines of the immediate stressors, allowing us to engage with life more fully.

Chapter 1: Foundation of Pranayama

In the vast landscape of yogic practices, Pranayama stands as a pillar of wisdom, offering seekers a profound gateway to self-discovery and well-being. This first chapter serves as a foundational exploration into the essence of Pranayama, laying the groundwork for a transformative journey into the art of conscious breathing.

1. The Breath as Life Force

At the heart of Pranayama lies a fundamental recognition—the breath is not merely a physiological process but a manifestation of a life force, known as prana. This section delves into the ancient understanding of prana and its role as the vital energy that animates our existence. We will explore the interconnected nature of breath, energy, and consciousness, setting the stage for the practices that follow.

2. Yogic Philosophy and Pranayama

Understanding Pranayama goes beyond the mechanical aspects of inhalation and exhalation; it is intricately woven into the fabric of yogic philosophy. This section provides insights into how Pranayama fits into the broader context of yoga, particularly as one of the eight limbs outlined by Patanjali in the Yoga Sutras. We will explore the philosophical underpinnings that guide the practice, emphasizing its role in achieving mental clarity and spiritual awakening.

3. Breath Awareness and Observation

Before delving into specific techniques, it is essential to cultivate an awareness of the breath. This segment introduces the practice of mindful breathing and breath observation. By becoming attuned to the natural rhythm of the breath, practitioners lay the groundwork for more advanced Pranayama techniques. The chapter will include practical exercises to enhance breath awareness in daily life.

4. The Three Pillars of Pranayama: Inhalation, Exhalation, and Retention

Pranayama involves conscious manipulation of the breath through three primary phases—inhalation, exhalation, and retention. This section breaks down each pillar, exploring their significance and the effects they have on the physical, mental, and energetic aspects of the practitioner. Techniques for developing control and mastery over each phase will be introduced.

5. Establishing a Pranayama Practice

To embark on a journey of transformation, consistency is key. This section provides practical guidance on establishing a sustainable and personalized Pranayama practice. From creating a conducive environment to setting realistic goals, practitioners will find insights on integrating Pranayama into their daily routines.

As we delve into the foundation of Pranayama, may this chapter serve as a compass, guiding you toward a deeper understanding of the breath as a gateway to profound well-being and self-discovery.

1.1 Ancient Wisdom and Modern Science

In the exploration of Pranayama, a captivating intersection emerges between the timeless wisdom of ancient traditions and the cutting-edge insights of modern science. This section delves into the symbiotic relationship between the ancient understanding of breath as a life force and the scientific revelations that validate and enhance our comprehension of the profound impact conscious breathing has on our well-being.

Ancient Wisdom: Prana as the Essence of Life

In the annals of ancient cultures, from the Vedic traditions of India to the practices of the Taoists in China, the concept of prana has held a central place. Prana, often referred to as the vital life force or cosmic energy, represents the animating principle that permeates all existence. It is within this ancient understanding that Pranayama finds its roots—the deliberate control and manipulation of prana through breath.

Modern Science: Unveiling the Mechanics of Breath

As science advances, so does our ability to unravel the intricacies of the human body and mind. Modern research corroborates the profound impact of conscious breathing on our physiological and psychological states. Studies demonstrate the influence of breath on the autonomic nervous system, hormonal balance, and cognitive function. This section delves into the scientific underpinnings of how Pranayama practices can directly affect heart rate variability, stress response, and overall mental well-being.

Harmony of Wisdom and Science: The Holistic Perspective

The convergence of ancient wisdom and modern science offers a holistic perspective on the significance of Pranayama. By acknowledging the intricate connection between breath, energy, and consciousness, we bridge the gap between the metaphysical and the measurable. This synthesis invites practitioners to approach Pranayama not only as a venerable tradition but as a validated and valuable tool for enhancing physical health, mental clarity, and emotional balance.

As we navigate the confluence of ancient wisdom and modern science, the journey into Pranayama becomes a harmonious blend of tradition and evidence-based practice. May this exploration inspire a deeper appreciation for the profound interplay between breath and well-being, transcending the boundaries of time and culture.

1.2 Breath Awareness Techniques

Before delving into the intricate practices of Pranayama, it is crucial to establish a strong foundation through breath awareness techniques. This section introduces methods to cultivate a mindful connection with the breath, laying the groundwork for a more profound exploration of conscious breathing.

1. Mindful Observation

The journey into breath awareness begins with the simple yet profound practice of mindful observation. In a quiet and comfortable space, take a few moments to sit or lie down. Direct your attention to the natural flow of your breath without attempting to control it. Observe the inhalation and exhalation, noticing the sensations, rhythm, and subtle pauses between breaths. This practice enhances present-moment awareness and sets the stage for more intentional breathwork.

2. Diaphragmatic Breathing

Also known as abdominal or belly breathing, diaphragmatic breathing focuses on engaging the diaphragm to facilitate a deeper breath. Place one hand on your chest and the other on your abdomen. Inhale slowly through your nose, allowing your abdomen to expand as the diaphragm descends. Exhale gently, feeling the abdomen contract. This technique encourages a more efficient and calming breath, promoting relaxation and reducing shallow chest breathing.

3. Box Breathing (Sama Vritti)

Box breathing, or Sama Vritti, is a structured breath awareness technique that involves equalizing the duration of inhalation, retention, exhalation, and another retention phase. Inhale to a count of four, hold the breath for four counts, exhale for four counts, and then maintain an empty lung state for another four counts. This rhythmic pattern fosters balance, mental focus, and a sense of calm.

4. Alternate Nostril Breathing (Nadi Shodhana)

Nadi Shodhana, or alternate nostril breathing, introduces the concept of balancing the flow of prana through the nostrils. Sitting comfortably, use the thumb and ring finger of the right hand to alternately close one nostril while inhaling and exhaling through the other. This technique harmonizes the left and right hemispheres of the brain, promoting mental clarity and energetic balance.

5. Full Yogic Breath

Full Yogic Breath involves a complete and conscious utilization of the lung capacity. Start by inhaling deeply through the nose, allowing the breath to fill the abdomen, diaphragm, and finally the chest. Exhale in the reverse order, emptying the chest, diaphragm, and abdomen. This practice enhances oxygenation, respiratory efficiency, and mindfulness of the entire breath cycle.

By incorporating these breath awareness techniques into your daily routine, you lay the groundwork for a more profound Pranayama practice. These simple yet potent exercises serve as a gateway to the transformative potential of conscious breathing, fostering a deeper connection between mind, body, and breath.

Chapter 2: Breath Control

In the exploration of Pranayama, the art of breath control takes center stage. Building upon the foundation laid in Chapter 1, this chapter delves into the intricacies of mastering the breath—exploring various techniques and principles that empower practitioners to regulate, refine, and harness the transformative potential of conscious breathing.

1. The Dynamics of Breath Control

Before embarking on specific breath control techniques, it is crucial to understand the dynamics at play. This section elucidates the relationship between breath control and the nervous system, highlighting how intentional regulation of the breath influences physiological responses. As practitioners grasp the connection between the breath and the body's subtle energies, they gain insight into the transformative power of conscious breath control.

2. Ujjayi Pranayama: The Victorious Breath

Ujjayi, often referred to as the "Victorious Breath" or "Ocean Breath," is a foundational technique in breath control. This section provides a detailed exploration of Ujjayi, characterized by the subtle contraction of the throat during both inhalation and exhalation. The resulting sound resembles the ocean waves, creating a soothing, rhythmic resonance. Ujjayi Pranayama enhances concentration, builds internal heat, and cultivates a sense of inner calm.

3. Kapalabhati: The Skull-Shining Breath

Kapalabhati, known as the "Skull-Shining Breath," involves rapid and forceful exhalations with passive inhalations. This dynamic technique cleanses the respiratory system, energizes the body, and stimulates the abdominal region. This section guides practitioners through the proper technique and gradual progression of Kapalabhati, emphasizing the importance of maintaining a steady and controlled pace.

4. Nadi Shodhana: Channel Purification

Building upon the breath awareness technique introduced earlier, Nadi Shodhana, or alternate nostril breathing, takes breath control to a deeper level. This section explores the balancing and purifying effects of Nadi Shodhana on the subtle energy channels (nadis) in the body. Practitioners learn precise hand positioning and breathe flow to synchronize the left and right hemispheres of the brain, promoting mental clarity and energetic harmony.

5. Bhramari Pranayama: The Humming Bee Breath

Bhramari Pranayama, or the "Humming Bee Breath," involves producing a gentle humming sound during exhalation. This section introduces the technique and explores its calming effects on the nervous system. Bhramari Pranayama is a valuable tool for stress reduction, promoting a tranquil mind and a heightened sense of inner awareness.

6. Advanced Breath Retention Techniques

This section explores advanced breath retention techniques, including Kumbhaka, or breath retention after inhalation or exhalation. As practitioners progress in their Pranayama journey, mastering these techniques enhances lung capacity, refines focus, and stimulates the flow of prana throughout the subtle energy channels.

7. Integrating Breath Control into Daily Life

Closing the chapter, this section provides insights into seamlessly integrating breath control practices into daily life. From mindful breathing during daily activities to incorporating specific techniques during moments of stress, practitioners discover the practical applications of breath control beyond the confines of a formal practice session.

As we delve into the realm of breath control, may this chapter serve as a guide, empowering practitioners to unlock the full potential of conscious breathing and its transformative effects on mind, body, and spirit.

2.1 Basics of Breath Control

Breath control, a fundamental aspect of Pranayama, involves the intentional regulation and refinement of the breath to influence both physiological and energetic states. Before delving into specific techniques, understanding the basics of breath control lays a crucial foundation for a more profound exploration of conscious breathing.

1. Awareness of the Breath

The journey into breath control begins with heightened awareness. Whether sitting in stillness or engaged in daily activities, cultivating mindfulness of the breath is the cornerstone. This awareness involves observing the natural rhythm of inhalation and exhalation without manipulation. By attuning to the breath's subtle nuances, practitioners establish a solid foundation for more intentional control.

2. Diaphragmatic Engagement

A key element in breath control is the engagement of the diaphragm. As the primary muscle of respiration, the diaphragm plays a vital role in facilitating deep, controlled breaths. Conscious diaphragmatic breathing involves allowing the diaphragm to descend on inhalation, expanding the abdomen, and ascending on exhalation, contracting the abdominal muscles. This simple yet powerful practice enhances respiratory efficiency and fosters a sense of calm.

3. Rhythmic Breathing

Breath control often revolves around establishing a steady and rhythmic pattern. This involves maintaining a consistent duration for both inhalation and exhalation. Beginners may start with a balanced ratio, gradually progressing to more intricate patterns. Rhythmic breathing promotes relaxation, balances the autonomic nervous system, and prepares the practitioner for more advanced techniques.

4. Posture and Alignment

The physical aspect of breath control is closely tied to posture and alignment. Whether sitting or standing, maintaining an upright spine and relaxed shoulders creates an optimal environment for unrestricted breathing. Proper alignment ensures the free flow of breath through the respiratory system, supporting the efficiency of breath control practices.

5. Gentle Transition into Breath Retention

As practitioners delve into breath control, a gentle introduction to breath retention becomes essential. This involves briefly pausing the breath after inhalation or exhalation, gradually increasing the duration as comfort and proficiency grow. Breath retention enhances lung capacity, refines focus, and prepares the respiratory system for more advanced Pranayama techniques.

6. Developing Patience and Consistency

Breath control is a skill that evolves with patience and consistent practice. Understanding that progress unfolds gradually allows practitioners to approach the journey with a sense of curiosity and openness. Regular, mindful engagement with breath control techniques deepens the connection between mind and breath, paving the way for a more profound exploration of Pranayama.

As practitioners master the basics of breath control, they establish a solid framework for the intricate techniques that follow. The simplicity of these foundational practices conceals a transformative power—an empowerment that extends beyond the mat into the tapestry of daily life. May the exploration of breath control be a harmonious step towards a more balanced and mindful existence.

2.2 Techniques for Lengthening and Deepening Breath

Breath, the subtle thread weaving through the fabric of life, holds the key to vitality and tranquility. In the realm of Pranayama, the ability to lengthen and deepen the breath is a cornerstone. This section explores techniques designed to expand the lung capacity, enhance oxygenation, and foster a profound connection between mind and breath.

1. Abdominal Breathing

Abdominal breathing, also known as diaphragmatic breathing, focuses on engaging the diaphragm to facilitate a deep inhalation. Place one hand on the chest and the other on the abdomen. Inhale slowly through the nose, allowing the abdomen to expand as the diaphragm descends. Exhale gently, feeling the abdomen contract. This technique enhances the utilization of the lower lungs, promoting a fuller breath and a sense of relaxation.

2. Three-Part Breath (Dirga Pranayama)

Dirga Pranayama, or the Three-Part Breath, involves sequential filling of the three parts of the lungs—lower, middle, and upper. Inhale deeply, allowing the breath to first fill the abdomen, then the chest, and finally reaching the upper lungs. Exhale in the reverse order. This technique promotes a complete breath cycle, maximizing oxygen intake and energizing the entire respiratory system.

3. Ratio Breathing

Ratio breathing involves consciously extending the duration of inhalation, exhalation, or both. Begin with a balanced ratio, such as inhaling for a count of four and exhaling for a count of four. Gradually experiment with different ratios, aiming for longer exhalations to enhance relaxation or longer inhalations for increased vitality. This technique refines breath control and encourages a mindful connection with the breath.

4. Ocean Breath (Ujjayi Pranayama)

Ujjayi Pranayama, often referred to as the Ocean Breath, involves a slight constriction of the throat during both inhalation and exhalation. This creates a subtle ocean-like sound, fostering concentration and depth in the breath. Inhale and exhale through the nose, allowing the breath to become both audible and soothing. Ujjayi Pranayama enhances breath awareness and encourages a more extended and controlled breath.

5. Extended Exhalation

A simple yet effective technique for deepening breath involves extending the exhalation phase. Inhale naturally, and then consciously lengthen the exhalation, allowing it to be twice as long as the inhalation. This practice activates the parasympathetic nervous system, promoting relaxation and reducing stress. Extended exhalation is a valuable tool for calming the mind and body.

6. Bellow Breath (Bhastrika Pranayama)

Bhastrika Pranayama, also known as Bellow Breath, involves forceful and rhythmic inhalations and exhalations through the nose. This dynamic technique expands lung capacity, invigorates the respiratory system, and increases oxygen intake. Practice Bhastrika with controlled intensity, gradually increasing the pace while maintaining awareness and steadiness.

By incorporating these techniques for lengthening and deepening the breath, practitioners embark on a journey of refining their respiratory capacity and enhancing the vital connection between breath and life. These practices not only enrich the experience of Pranayama but also serve as valuable tools for cultivating a harmonious and balanced existence.

Chapter 3: The Power of Breath

In the intricate tapestry of Pranayama, Chapter 3 explores the profound influence and transformative potential inherent in the power of breath. As we delve deeper into the practices, philosophies, and physiological aspects, this chapter unfolds the layers of understanding that illuminate the breath as a catalyst for holistic well-being.

1. The Breath-Mind Connection

Central to the power of breath is its undeniable connection to the mind. This section explores the intricate interplay between breath and mental states. Through conscious breath control, practitioners gain insights into managing stress, enhancing focus, and cultivating emotional resilience. The breath becomes a bridge, linking the external world to the inner landscape of thoughts and emotions.

2. Prana: The Energetic Essence

At the heart of Pranayama lies the concept of prana—an expansive force that permeates the cosmos and flows within each living being. This section delves into the ancient wisdom that views breathe as the carrier of prana, connecting the physical body to the subtle energies. Understanding prana unveils the deeper layers of the breath's influence on vitality, clarity, and the balance of the energetic body.

3. Breath and Stress Resilience

In the modern whirlwind of stress, the breath emerges as a powerful ally. Techniques for stress reduction through Pranayama are explored, emphasizing the role of conscious breathing in modulating the body's stress response. This section introduces practices to induce a state of calm, balance cortisol levels, and foster resilience in the face of life's challenges.

4. Mindfulness and Presence

Mindfulness, rooted in breath awareness, becomes a gateway to living in the present moment. This section unravels the transformative impact of mindful breathing on daily life. As practitioners learn to anchor their awareness in the breath, they cultivate a heightened state of presence that transcends the chaos of the external world, fostering a profound sense of peace and clarity.

5. Breath and Physical Well-Being

Beyond its impact on the mind, the breath plays a pivotal role in physical well-being. This section explores the physiological benefits of Pranayama, including enhanced lung capacity, improved oxygenation, and the promotion of cardiovascular health. Breath control becomes a tool for optimizing the body's functions, supporting overall vitality and resilience.

6. The Meditative Breath

As practitioners advance in their Pranayama journey, the breath evolves into a meditative instrument. This section introduces contemplative practices that harness the meditative power of the breath. Through techniques such as breath observation and silent breath counting, practitioners deepen their connection to the inner self, unraveling the layers of consciousness.

7. Integrating the Power of Breath into Life

Closing the chapter, we explore the practical integration of the power of breath into daily life. From mindful breathing in mundane activities to incorporating specific Pranayama techniques during challenging moments, practitioners discover how the breath becomes a constant source of renewal, resilience, and joy.

In Chapter 3, the power of breath unfolds as a multifaceted gem, offering insights into the interconnected realms of mind, energy, and physical well-being. May this exploration inspire practitioners to embrace the transformative potential of conscious breathing, unlocking the gates to a harmonious and enriched existence.

3.1 Harnessing Energy through Pranayama

In the expansive realm of Pranayama, the practice becomes a dynamic conduit for harnessing energy—both physical and subtle. This section unravels the intricacies of how conscious breathing, as a vehicle for prana, empowers practitioners to tap into a wellspring of vitality, mental clarity, and spiritual insight.

1. Prana: The Essence of Life

Prana, often described as the life force or vital energy, is the animating essence that courses through the universe and every living being. This subsection delves into the foundational understanding of prana as the driving force behind the breath, exploring its connection to the body, mind, and the broader energetic system. By recognizing prana as the subtle thread woven into the breath, practitioners embark on a journey to consciously channel and amplify this vital energy.

2. Breath as a Conduit for Prana

The breath serves as the primary vehicle for prana, carrying this life force into every cell of the body. Here, we explore how intentional breath control, practiced through various Pranayama techniques, allows individuals to regulate the flow of prana. By refining the breath, practitioners gain mastery over the energetic currents within, unlocking the transformative potential of prana in promoting holistic well-being.

3. Vitality and Mental Clarity

Conscious engagement with Pranayama becomes a means to infuse the body and mind with vitality. Through specific breath control techniques, practitioners enhance oxygenation, optimize respiratory function, and invigorate the body's energy systems. This heightened vitality extends to the mental realm, promoting mental clarity, focus, and heightened awareness. The breath, as a carrier of prana, becomes a source of sustainable energy that nourishes both body and mind.

4. Balancing Energy Centers (Chakras)

The yogic tradition posits the existence of energy centers known as chakras, each associated with specific qualities and aspects of consciousness. This subsection explores how Pranayama acts as a tool to balance and activate these energy centers. By directing the breath with intention, practitioners harmonize the flow of prana, fostering a sense of equilibrium and well-being across the physical and energetic dimensions of the self.

5. Awakening Spiritual Insight

As practitioners deepen their exploration of Pranayama, the breath becomes a gateway to heightened spiritual insight. This section delves into the meditative aspects of breath control, where the practice transcends the physical and energetic realms to touch the spiritual core. Through techniques that cultivate stillness and profound awareness, individuals unlock the door to spiritual awakening and a deeper connection to the universal source of prana.

6. The Integration of Prana into Life

Closing this exploration, we delve into the practical integration of prana harnessing techniques into daily life. From energizing morning routines to mindful breath breaks throughout the day, practitioners discover how the conscious cultivation and utilization of prana become a transformative and sustainable practice, enriching every facet of their existence.

In harnessing energy through Pranayama, practitioners embark on a journey that transcends the boundaries of the physical and ushers them into the expansive realms of vitality, clarity, and spiritual awakening. May this understanding inspire a harmonious integration of prana into daily life, fostering a life imbued with vibrant energy and profound insight.

3.2 Connecting Breath and Emotions

In the intricate dance of the mind and body, the breath serves as a bridge between the conscious and the subconscious, connecting intimately with our emotional landscape. This section explores how the artful practice of Pranayama weaves a profound connection between breath and emotions, offering practitioners a transformative tool for emotional well-being and self-awareness.

1. The Breath-Emotion Nexus

The breath and emotions share an intricate relationship—each influencing the other in a continuous feedback loop. This subsection delves into the physiological and psychological dimensions of this connection. As emotions arise, they manifest in the breath—shallow during stress, deep in moments of calm. Conversely, intentional breath control becomes a means to modulate and regulate the intensity and quality of emotions.

2. Breath as an Emotional Barometer

Pranayama practices teach practitioners to regard the breath as an ever-present emotional barometer. By observing the breath during different emotional states, individuals gain insights into their inner landscape. This heightened awareness allows for the recognition of emotions as they surface and provides an opportunity to navigate them with mindfulness.

3. Calming the Emotional Storm

In moments of emotional turbulence, the breath becomes a steadfast anchor. Techniques that emphasize slow, deep breaths, such as diaphragmatic breathing, soothe the nervous system and promote emotional equilibrium. This section introduces specific Pranayama practices aimed at calming the sympathetic nervous system, fostering relaxation, and providing a sanctuary amidst emotional storms.

4. Releasing Emotional Blockages

Pranayama serves as a powerful tool for releasing emotional blockages stored in the body. Techniques that involve deep inhalations and full exhalations facilitate the release of pent-up emotions, allowing practitioners to experience a sense of emotional release and catharsis. This process enables individuals to cultivate emotional resilience and move towards a more balanced state.

5. Emotional Intelligence and Mindful Breathing

Mindful breath awareness becomes a catalyst for emotional intelligence. This subsection explores how the regular practice of observing the breath without judgment enhances emotional self-awareness. As practitioners develop a mindful relationship with their breath, they gain the capacity to respond to emotions with greater discernment and compassion.

6. Breathwork for Emotional Expression

Certain Pranayama techniques encourage conscious emotional expression. Through practices that involve vocalization, such as Bhramari Pranayama (the Humming Bee Breath), individuals have the means to release and express emotions in a controlled and intentional manner. This section illuminates how these practices can serve as therapeutic tools for emotional well-being.

7. Cultivating Positive Emotional States

Pranayama offers avenues to intentionally cultivate positive emotional states. Techniques that emphasize heart-centered breathing or emphasize joyous inhalations can uplift the emotional state. By consciously choosing breath patterns that align with desired emotional experiences, practitioners harness the transformative potential of breath to create a positive emotional tapestry.

As we explore the profound connection between breath and emotions, Pranayama emerges as an artful navigation tool through the intricate landscape of human feelings. May this understanding empower practitioners to cultivate emotional resilience, self-awareness, and a harmonious relationship with their emotional selves through the intentional dance with breath.

Chapter 4: Mind-Body Connection

In the holistic journey of Pranayama, Chapter 4 illuminates the intricate interplay between the mind and body. This symbiotic relationship forms the essence of the practice, transcending the physical breath to delve into the realms of mental clarity, emotional balance, and overall well-being.

1. The Mind-Body Nexus

At the heart of Pranayama lies the profound connection between the mind and body. This section explores how the breath serves as a subtle but potent link, influencing the intricate dance of thoughts, emotions, and physical sensations. The mind-body nexus becomes the canvas upon which practitioners paint the art of conscious breathing.

2. Breath as a Mirror of the Mind

The breath mirrors the state of the mind, and vice versa. This subsection delves into the concept that the qualities of the breath—whether calm or agitated—reflect the mental landscape. By observing the breath, practitioners gain insights into the ever-changing currents of the mind, fostering a deeper understanding of their mental states.

3. Conscious Breath, Conscious Mind

Pranayama becomes a gateway to conscious living—a practice that extends mindfulness to every breath. This section explores how intentional breath control refines awareness and presence. As practitioners engage with the breath consciously, the mind follows suit, entering a state of heightened awareness that transcends the confines of routine thought patterns.

4. The Influence of Breath on Stress Response

The mind-body connection is particularly poignant in the modulation of the stress response. This subsection delves into the impact of conscious breathing on the autonomic nervous system. Through specific Pranayama techniques, practitioners learn to navigate the delicate balance between the sympathetic and parasympathetic branches, fostering resilience and calming the stress response.

5. Enhancing Cognitive Function

Pranayama emerges as a cognitive enhancer, sharpening mental faculties and improving cognitive function. Techniques that involve focused attention on the breath, such as mindfulness-based practices, stimulate the brain's executive functions. This section explores how the intentional regulation of breath becomes a tool for improving concentration, memory, and overall cognitive performance.

6. Breath and Emotional Regulation

The mind-body connection extends to emotional regulation. Pranayama becomes an emotional alchemist, offering practitioners the means to navigate and modulate emotional states. This subsection introduces specific breath control practices that foster emotional balance, equipping individuals with tools to respond to emotions with mindfulness and resilience.

7. The Role of Breath in Physical Well-Being

Beyond mental and emotional realms, the mind-body connection significantly impacts physical well-being. This section explores how Pranayama contributes to physical health, including enhanced lung capacity, improved cardiovascular function, and overall vitality. The breath becomes a vehicle for optimizing the body's functions and supporting holistic health.

8. Integrating Mind-Body Awareness into Daily Life

Closing the chapter, we explore the practical integration of mind-body awareness into daily life. From mindful breathing in routine activities to conscious pauses during moments of stress, practitioners discover how the intentional alignment of mind and body through breath becomes a foundation for a balanced and enriched existence.

In Chapter 4, the mind-body connection unfolds as a tapestry woven with every conscious breath. May this exploration inspire practitioners to cultivate a harmonious union between mind and body, fostering a state of well-being that permeates every facet of their lives.

4.1 Balancing the Mind through Breath

In the intricate symphony of the mind and body, Pranayama emerges as a profound conductor, orchestrating harmony through conscious breath. This section delves into the art of balancing the mind through intentional breath control, exploring how the breath becomes a nuanced instrument for cultivating mental equilibrium.

1. Breath as a Mirror of the Mind

The breath, like a reflective surface, mirrors the ever-shifting landscape of the mind. This subsection illuminates the symbiotic relationship between the quality of the breath and mental states. By keenly observing the breath, practitioners gain insights into the fluctuations of the mind—calm breaths echoing serenity, agitated breaths mirroring unrest. Recognizing this mirror-like connection becomes the first step in the journey to balance the mind.

2. Mindful Breath Awareness

Balancing the mind begins with mindful breath awareness. The practice involves observing the breath without judgment, bringing attention to the present moment. This mindful awareness serves as a foundation, allowing practitioners to disentangle from the whirlwind of thoughts and emotions, fostering a serene and focused mental landscape.

3. Regulating Stress Response

Pranayama becomes a potent tool in regulating the stress response, ushering the mind into a state of equilibrium. Techniques that emphasize slow, deep breaths activate the parasympathetic nervous system, counteracting the effects of stress. This section explores how intentional breath control acts as a calming force, promoting mental resilience in the face of life's challenges.

4. Cultivating Emotional Balance

The breath, as an intimate companion to emotions, becomes a guide in cultivating emotional balance. Through specific Pranayama practices, practitioners learn to navigate and modulate emotional states. Techniques that involve extended exhalations or alternate nostril breathing foster emotional equilibrium, empowering individuals to respond to emotions with mindfulness and composure.

5. Harnessing Breath for Concentration

Concentration is a hallmark of a balanced mind, and Pranayama serves as a vehicle for sharpening this faculty. This subsection explores techniques that involve focused attention on the breath, such as mindfulness-based practices. By engaging the mind in the rhythmic flow of the breath, practitioners enhance concentration, clarity of thought, and the ability to remain present in the current moment.

6. Quieting the Mental Chatter

The mind often becomes a cacophony of thoughts, drowning out the stillness within. Pranayama acts as a gentle conductor, quieting the mental chatter. Techniques like Ujjayi Pranayama, with its soothing sound resembling ocean waves, guide practitioners into a state of mental calmness. The breath becomes a rhythmic melody that leads the mind into a serene and centered space.

7. Integrating Breath Balance into Life

Closing this exploration, we delve into the practical integration of breath balance into daily life. From incorporating mindful breathing into daily routines to taking intentional breath breaks during hectic moments, practitioners discover how the breath becomes a reliable anchor in navigating the ebb and flow of the mind. The balanced breath serves as a compass, guiding individuals toward mental clarity and serenity.

In the realm of Pranayama, balancing the mind through breath is not just a practice; it is an art—a dance that harmonizes the rhythms of the breath with the melodies of the mind. May this understanding empower practitioners to embrace the transformative potential of conscious breathing, fostering a balanced and serene state of mind.

4.2 Enhancing Physical Well-being

Pranayama, the ancient art of breath control, transcends the boundaries of the mind and extends its transformative touch to the physical realm. This section explores how conscious breathing becomes a powerful catalyst for enhancing physical well-being, optimizing the body's functions, and fostering vitality.

1. Oxygenation and Respiratory Efficiency

At the core of physical well-being lies the fundamental process of oxygenation. Pranayama techniques, such as deep diaphragmatic breathing, enhance the efficiency of oxygen exchange in the lungs. This subsection delves into how intentional breath control improves respiratory function, increasing the oxygen supply to cells and tissues, and promoting overall vitality.

2. Lung Capacity and Respiratory Health

Pranayama serves as a bespoke workout for the respiratory system, strengthening lung capacity and promoting respiratory health. Techniques that involve full, deep breaths—such as Full Yogic Breath—expand the lungs' capacity. This section explores how the deliberate regulation of breath optimizes respiratory mechanics, fostering resilience and supporting the body's natural ability to ward off respiratory ailments.

3. Cardiovascular Benefits

The breath, as a rhythmic conductor, influences the cardiovascular system. Through specific Pranayama practices, practitioners engage in a dynamic interplay that benefits heart health. Techniques like Bhastrika Pranayama, with its invigorating breath pattern, stimulate circulation, improve blood flow, and support cardiovascular well-being. This subsection explores the profound connection between intentional breath control and a healthy heart.

4. Stress Reduction and Immune Support

The physical toll of stress on the body is significant, impacting the immune system. Pranayama emerges as a powerful ally in stress reduction, calming the nervous system and mitigating the effects of chronic stress. By fostering a state of relaxation through intentional breath control, practitioners support immune function, enhancing the body's resilience against illness.

5. Digestive Harmony through Breath

The breath extends its influence to the digestive system, contributing to digestive harmony. Techniques that emphasize diaphragmatic breathing and breath awareness, when practiced mindfully, stimulate the parasympathetic nervous system. This promotes optimal digestion, absorption of nutrients, and overall gut health. This subsection explores the intricate connection between breath and digestive well-being.

6. Muscular Relaxation and Flexibility

Pranayama becomes a gateway to muscular relaxation and enhanced flexibility. Through breath control, practitioners induce a state of calmness that extends to the muscular system. Techniques like Nadi Shodhana, with its balancing effects, promote flexibility and release muscular tension. This section explores how intentional breath practices contribute to overall physical suppleness and well-being.

7. Integrating Breath into Physical Activities

Closing the exploration, we delve into the practical integration of breath practices into physical activities. Whether during exercise, yoga asanas, or daily movement, conscious breathing becomes a guiding force. This integration not only enhances the efficacy of physical endeavors but also transforms routine activities into mindful practices, fostering a holistic approach to physical well-being.

In the journey of Pranayama, the enhancement of physical well-being through breath is not a mere side effect but a deliberate and transformative process. May this understanding inspire practitioners to embrace the holistic benefits of conscious breathing, nurturing a resilient and vibrant foundation for their physical health and well-being.

Chapter 5: Spirituality and Pranayama

As we ascend the peaks of Pranayama, Chapter 5 invites us into the transcendent realms of spirituality. Beyond the physical and mental dimensions, the breath becomes a sacred bridge connecting the individual soul to the universal essence. This chapter explores how the practice of Pranayama becomes a transformative journey into the heart of spirituality.

1. The Breath as Spiritual Essence

In the spiritual tapestry, the breath is revered as more than a physiological process—it is the essence of life itself. This section delves into the ancient wisdom that recognizes the breath as a divine force, carrying the spark of the eternal. As practitioners engage in conscious breathing, they embark on a journey to rediscover the spiritual essence within every breath.

2. Pranayama as a Spiritual Practice

Pranayama transcends its role as a physical and mental practice to become a sacred discipline. This subsection explores how the intentional regulation of breath becomes a spiritual offering—an act of devotion that aligns the individual with the cosmic rhythms. Through breath, practitioners cultivate a profound sense of presence, connecting to the divine within and around them.

3. Breath and Meditation: Bridging the Inner Silence

Meditation and Pranayama intertwine as kindred practices on the spiritual path. This section illuminates how conscious breath control serves as a bridge to inner silence. Techniques such as breath observation and mindful breathing pave the way for a meditative state, where the mind becomes a tranquil lake reflecting the boundless expanses of spiritual consciousness.

4. Awakening the Kundalini Energy

In the yogic tradition, the awakening of Kundalini energy is a pivotal aspect of spiritual evolution. This subsection explores how specific Pranayama techniques act as catalysts for awakening and channeling this potent spiritual force. The breath, as a vehicle for prana, becomes the sacred river that nourishes the dormant serpent energy at the base of the spine.

5. The Subtle Energy Channels: Nadi Shodhana

Nadi Shodhana, or alternate nostril breathing, takes center stage as a gateway to spiritual awakening. This section delves into how this practice purifies and balances the subtle energy channels (nadis) in the body. As practitioners navigate the rhythmic flow of breath through alternate nostrils, they harmonize the dual forces within, paving the way for spiritual integration.

6. Surrendering in Breath Control

Spirituality often invites the practice of surrender—a letting go of the egoic self. In Pranayama, practitioners discover the transformative power of surrendering in breath control. This subsection explores how the conscious release of control over the breath becomes a symbolic act of surrender, opening the door to spiritual humility and receptivity.

7. Breath and Sound: Mantra in Pranayama

Sound, intertwined with breath, becomes a sacred medium in Pranayama. This section explores the integration of mantra—the vibrational essence of sound—into breath practices. Through the rhythmic chanting of sacred sounds, practitioners infuse their breath with spiritual resonance, elevating the practice to a meditative and devotional expression.

8. Living the Spiritual Breath

Closing the chapter, we explore the practical integration of spiritual breath into daily life. From mindfulness in ordinary activities to intentional breath breaks as acts of reverence, practitioners learn to infuse every moment with the sanctity of the spiritual breath. This integration becomes a living expression of spirituality, weaving the sacred thread of breath through the fabric of existence.

In Chapter 5, Pranayama unfolds as a sacred journey into spirituality—a pilgrimage guided by the breath. May this exploration inspire practitioners to traverse the realms of the divine within, unlocking the gates to profound spiritual awakening and a harmonious union with the universal essence.

5.1 Deepening the Spiritual Practice

Within the sacred corridors of Pranayama, the breath transforms into a vessel that carries practitioners into the depths of spiritual exploration. This section unravels the nuances of deepening the spiritual practice, delving into the mystical realms where the breath becomes a sacred thread connecting the individual soul to the vastness of the spiritual landscape.

1. The Sacred Breath Essence

At the heart of deepening the spiritual practice lies the recognition of the breath as a sacred essence. This subsection illuminates the profound understanding that each breath carries the divine spark—the very essence that connects the individual to the universal source of all existence. Practitioners embark on a journey to attune themselves to this sacred breath, realizing it as a continuous communion with the spiritual realm.

2. Rituals of Conscious Breathing

The practice of conscious breathing transcends routine—it becomes a sacred ritual. This section explores how practitioners infuse intention and reverence into each breath, transforming the act of breathing into a ritualistic communion with the divine. By bringing mindfulness to the rhythm, depth, and intention of each breath, individuals create a sacred space where the spiritual essence is invoked.

3. Breath as a Prayer

In the deepening of the spiritual practice, the breath evolves into a prayer—a silent communication with the divine. This subsection explores how conscious breathing becomes a sacred language, expressing devotion, gratitude, and surrender. As practitioners breathe with intention, each inhale and exhale becomes a whispered prayer, echoing through the chambers of the soul.

4. The Stillness Between Breaths

The spaces between breaths hold a mystical quality—an invitation to the realm of stillness. This section delves into the practice of embracing the silence between breaths, where the mind transcends ordinary thought and connects with the divine silence within. Practitioners navigate this sacred stillness, attuning themselves to the timeless presence that exists beyond the rhythmic dance of inhalation and exhalation.

5. Breath and Spiritual Mindfulness

Spiritual mindfulness unfolds as practitioners bring a heightened awareness to the breath in every moment. This subsection explores how mindfulness expands beyond formal practices, infusing every aspect of life with spiritual presence. Whether in mundane activities or moments of challenge, individuals learn to carry the sacred breath into each experience, fostering a continuous connection with the divine.

6. Surrendering the Ego in Breath

Deepening the spiritual practice involves a profound surrender—an offering of the egoic self to the divine flow. This section explores the transformative power of surrendering the ego in breath control. As practitioners release the need for control and let the breath guide them, they enter a state of humility and openness, allowing the divine essence to permeate their being.

7. Breath as a Path to Self-Realization

The spiritual journey is a path of self-realization, and the breath becomes a guiding light. This subsection explores how conscious breathing leads practitioners to a deeper understanding of the self—a realization of the eternal essence beyond the transient layers of identity. The breath, as a companion on this path, unveils the truth that the individual soul is inseparable from the universal soul.

8. Integration of Spiritual Breath in Daily Life

Closing the exploration, we delve into the integration of the spiritual breath into daily life. From mindful breath breaks to infusing ordinary activities with sacred awareness, practitioners learn to live the spiritual breath continuously. This integration becomes a living expression of the divine within, weaving the sacred thread of breath through the fabric of existence.

In the profound depths of spiritual practice, the breath unveils its mystical nature, becoming a transformative force that leads practitioners to the core of their spiritual being. May this exploration inspire a deepening commitment to the sacred journey within, where each breath becomes a prayer and every moment an expression of divine communion.

5.2 Exploring Higher States of Consciousness

Within the boundless realms of Pranayama, practitioners embark on a sacred quest to explore higher states of consciousness. In this transcendent journey, the breath becomes a mystical guide, leading individuals beyond the ordinary realms of perception into the luminous expanses of spiritual awakening.

1. The Breath as a Gateway to the Divine

At the threshold of higher consciousness, the breath stands as a sacred gateway. This subsection illuminates how practitioners, through conscious breath control, open this gateway to the divine. The breath becomes a subtle bridge connecting the individual soul to the cosmic consciousness, inviting a journey into dimensions beyond ordinary perception.

2. Transcending Ordinary Awareness

Higher states of consciousness transcend the limitations of ordinary awareness. This section explores how specific Pranayama practices, such as extended breath retention and rhythmic breath modulation, serve as keys to unlocking the doors to expanded states of perception. Practitioners navigate the subtle currents of breath to access realms where the mind transcends its usual boundaries.

3. Breathwork and Altered States of Perception

Breathwork becomes a vehicle for navigating altered states of perception. This subsection delves into how intentional breath control induces altered states, unlocking doorways to heightened intuition, expanded awareness, and profound spiritual experiences. Through breath, practitioners traverse the landscapes of consciousness, unveiling the infinite potential within.

4. The Role of Prana in Consciousness Expansion

Prana, the life force carried by the breath, becomes the key player in the expansion of consciousness. This section explores the relationship between prana and consciousness, emphasizing how conscious breath control allows individuals to channel and amplify this vital force. Through the refinement of pranic flow, practitioners elevate their consciousness to transcendent realms.

5. Kundalini Awakening and Conscious Breath

Kundalini, the dormant spiritual energy, unfolds through conscious breath practices. This subsection delves into how specific Pranayama techniques act as catalysts for the awakening of Kundalini. As the breath becomes a vehicle for the pranic ascent, practitioners witness the profound transformation that accompanies the rising of this sacred energy, leading to heightened states of awareness.

6. Breath and Spiritual Vision

The breath, when harnessed with intention, becomes a conduit for spiritual vision. This section explores how practices like Trataka, or focused gazing, integrated with conscious breathing, elevate visual perception to spiritual heights. Practitioners embark on a journey where the eyes become windows to the soul, revealing the luminosity within.

7. Silence as the Ultimate Breath

In the exploration of higher consciousness, silence becomes the ultimate breath. This subsection illuminates how the stillness between breaths and the cultivation of inner silence lead practitioners to the core of spiritual awakening. Through practices that emphasize the tranquil breath, individuals touch the timeless essence beyond the realm of words and thoughts.

8. Living in Transcendent Consciousness

Closing the exploration, we delve into the integration of transcendent consciousness into daily life. From carrying the awareness of higher states into routine activities to radiating the peace of expanded consciousness in interactions, practitioners learn to live in the world while anchored in the transcendent. The breath becomes the constant companion, guiding individuals to navigate the dual dance of the spiritual and material realms.

In the sacred exploration of higher states of consciousness, the breath unfolds its mystical potential, inviting practitioners to soar beyond the boundaries of ordinary perception. May this journey into the realms of expanded awareness inspire a profound spiritual awakening, where each breath becomes a step into the luminous landscapes of the divine.

Chapter 6: Integrating Pranayama into Daily Life

As the transformative journey of Pranayama unfolds, Chapter 6 serves as a guide to seamlessly weave the wisdom of conscious breathing into the fabric of everyday existence. This chapter explores practical ways to integrate Pranayama into daily life, fostering a harmonious alignment between breath, mind, and spirit.

1. Breath as the Anchor in Routine

In the tapestry of daily routines, the breath emerges as a steadfast anchor. This section illuminates how conscious breathing can be seamlessly integrated into the rhythm of daily life. From mindful breath breaks during work to infusing awareness into mundane tasks, practitioners discover how the breath becomes a guiding force, fostering a sense of presence and calm amidst the busyness of routine.

2. Morning Rituals for Mindful Beginnings

The start of the day holds the potential for intentional beginnings. This subsection explores morning rituals infused with Pranayama practices, setting the tone for a mindful and centered day. Whether through breath-awareness meditation or energizing breath techniques, individuals cultivate a sacred space in the early hours, aligning their breath with the promise of a harmonious day ahead.

3. Breath Breaks for Stressful Moments

In the face of stress and challenges, breath breaks become potent tools for resilience. This section delves into the practice of turning to conscious breathing during moments of tension. Techniques for quick, calming breaths empower individuals to navigate stress with grace, fostering emotional balance and preventing the accumulation of tension in the body and mind.

4. Breath in Mindful Movement

Physical movement becomes a canvas for breath awareness. This subsection explores how Pranayama seamlessly integrates into mindful movement practices, such as yoga or tai chi. By synchronizing breath with movement, individuals enhance the mind-body connection, fostering a sense of fluidity, grace, and meditative presence in every step and posture.

5. Breathing Through Work and Productivity

The workplace, often a realm of constant activity, becomes an arena for conscious breath engagement. This section explores how practitioners can incorporate breath practices into work routines to enhance focus, creativity, and productivity. From conscious breathing during breaks to using specific techniques for mental clarity, individuals optimize their work environment through the transformative power of breath.

6. Evening Practices for Relaxation

As the day winds down, Pranayama becomes a gateway to relaxation and rejuvenation. This subsection explores evening practices that invite individuals to unwind through breath. Techniques emphasizing slow, deep breaths or calming breath patterns prepare the mind and body for restful sleep, promoting a sense of tranquility as the day concludes.

7. Mindful Eating and Breath Connection

Eating transforms into a mindful ritual when paired with conscious breathing. This section delves into the practice of cultivating breath awareness during meals. By slowing down the pace of eating and synchronizing breath with each bite, individuals enhance digestion, promote mindful nourishment, and foster a deeper connection with the act of eating as a sacred process.

8. Nighttime Reflection and Breath

Before embracing the stillness of the night, individuals can turn to breath practices for reflection and introspection. This subsection explores nighttime rituals that involve conscious breathing. From breath-awareness meditation to gratitude practices, practitioners create a sacred space for self-reflection, fostering a sense of peace and gratitude as they transition into the realm of dreams.

In Chapter 6, Pranayama seamlessly integrates into the tapestry of daily life, offering a guiding thread that weaves through each moment. May this exploration inspire practitioners to infuse their days with the wisdom of conscious breathing, creating a harmonious dance between breath and life, spirit and routine.

6.1 Creating a Personal Practice

Embarking on a journey of integration, this section delves into the art of crafting a personalized Pranayama practice—a sacred space where breath becomes a companion in daily life. By tailoring the practice to individual needs and preferences, practitioners cultivate a harmonious relationship with breath, fostering a sense of well-being and mindfulness.

1. Understanding Personal Intentions

Creating a personal Pranayama practice begins with understanding individual intentions. This subsection guides practitioners to reflect on their goals—whether seeking relaxation, stress reduction, increased energy, or spiritual connection. By clarifying intentions, individuals lay the foundation for a practice that aligns with their unique needs and aspirations.

2. Choosing Appropriate Techniques

Personalized Pranayama practices are crafted by selecting techniques that resonate with individual preferences. This section introduces a variety of techniques—ranging from calming breaths like Nadi Shodhana to energizing practices like Kapalabhati. Practitioners are encouraged to explore and experiment, selecting techniques that harmonize with their physical, mental, and spiritual inclinations.

3. Establishing a Consistent Routine

Consistency is key to cultivating the transformative benefits of Pranayama. This subsection guides individuals in establishing a routine tailored to their lifestyle. Whether incorporating breath practices into morning rituals or dedicating specific times for breath breaks throughout the day, a consistent routine becomes the scaffold upon which the personalized practice unfolds.

4. Adapting to Changing Needs

The dynamic nature of life calls for adaptability in one's practice. This section encourages practitioners to be attuned to changing needs and circumstances. Whether adjusting the duration of the practice, incorporating different techniques, or adapting to evolving intentions, flexibility ensures that the personalized practice remains a fluid and responsive tool for well-being.

5. Mindful Breath Journaling

Journaling becomes a companion in the journey of personal practice. This subsection introduces the practice of mindful breath journaling—documenting experiences, reflections, and observations after each session.

Through journaling, individuals gain insights into the evolving relationship with breath, deepening their understanding and enhancing the potency of the practice.

6. Integrating Breath with Mindfulness

A personalized Pranayama practice intertwines seamlessly with mindfulness. This section explores the integration of breath awareness into everyday activities. Practitioners are encouraged to bring mindful breathing into moments of work, relaxation, and connection, allowing the practice to permeate all aspects of daily life.

7. Seeking Guidance and Progression

The journey of creating a personal Pranayama practice benefits from guidance and progression. This subsection emphasizes the importance of seeking guidance from experienced teachers or resources, especially for those new to breathwork. Additionally, individuals are encouraged to progress gradually, respecting the body's signals and gradually deepening their practice over time.

8. Cultivating Joy in the Practice

In the tapestry of a personal Pranayama practice, joy becomes a vital thread. This section invites practitioners to infuse joy into their breathwork. Whether through exploring new techniques, celebrating milestones, or savoring the moments of stillness, joy becomes a transformative energy that nourishes the soul on the journey of conscious breathing.

In creating a personal Pranayama practice, individuals embark on a unique and sacred journey—one that unfolds in alignment with their intentions, needs, and the ever-changing rhythms of life. May this exploration inspire practitioners to weave a tapestry of breath that brings balance, vitality, and mindful presence into every moment of their daily lives.

6.2 Overcoming Challenges and Establishing Consistency

While the path of Pranayama offers profound benefits, it is not immune to challenges that may arise on the journey. In this section, we explore strategies for overcoming obstacles and establishing the consistency that is fundamental to reaping the transformative rewards of conscious breathwork.

1. Identifying Common Challenges

Understanding the common challenges that may surface in a Pranayama practice is the first step towards overcoming them. This subsection sheds light on challenges such as distractions, restlessness, physical discomfort, or time constraints. By recognizing these hurdles, practitioners gain awareness and set the stage for effective solutions.

2. Creating a Supportive Environment

Establishing a supportive environment is crucial for consistency. This section guides individuals to create a space conducive to their breath practice—free from distractions, comfortable, and infused with a sense of tranquility. By dedicating a specific area for breathwork, practitioners enhance focus and invite a harmonious atmosphere into their practice.

3. Time Management and Prioritization

Time constraints often pose a challenge in maintaining consistency. This subsection explores strategies for effective time management, encouraging practitioners to prioritize their breath practice. By allocating dedicated time slots and viewing the practice as a non-negotiable part of the day, individuals weave a thread of regularity into the fabric of their routine.

4. Adapting Practices to Fit Schedule

Flexibility in adapting practices to fit one's schedule is a key element of overcoming challenges. This section introduces the concept of short, effective breath sessions that can be seamlessly integrated into busy days. Whether through micro-practices or incorporating breath awareness into daily tasks, practitioners learn to adapt the practice to the ebb and flow of their lives.

5. Cultivating Mindfulness Amidst Distractions

Distractions can derail even the most dedicated practice. This subsection explores techniques for cultivating mindfulness amidst distractions. By acknowledging external disruptions without judgment and gently redirecting focus to the breath, individuals build resilience against distractions, fostering a sense of presence and concentration.

6. Addressing Physical Discomfort

Physical discomfort, whether due to posture or breath techniques, can be a hindrance. This section provides insights into addressing and mitigating physical discomfort. From exploring alternative postures to adjusting the intensity of breath practices, practitioners learn to listen to their bodies and adapt the practice for comfort and sustainability.

7. Leveraging Technology for Support

In the digital age, technology can be a valuable ally in maintaining consistency. This subsection explores the use of apps, guided sessions, or online communities for support and motivation. By leveraging technology mindfully, practitioners can enhance their connection to the practice and tap into a virtual community for encouragement.

8. Celebrating Progress and Milestones

Celebrating progress, no matter how small, becomes a powerful motivator. This section encourages practitioners to acknowledge milestones in their Pranayama journey. Whether it's mastering a challenging technique or sustaining a consistent practice, celebrating achievements creates a positive feedback loop, nurturing enthusiasm and commitment.

By navigating and overcoming challenges, practitioners lay a resilient foundation for their Pranayama practice. Consistency, rooted in mindful adaptation and perseverance, becomes the bridge between challenges and the transformative benefits of conscious breathwork. May this exploration empower individuals to cultivate a consistent and enriching relationship with their breath, fostering well-being and mindfulness.

Chapter 7: Breathwork for Harmonious Living

In the culmination of our exploration, Chapter 7 delves into the profound integration of breathwork into the tapestry of everyday life. Breath becomes not merely a practice but a guiding force for harmonious living—nurturing well-being, fostering mindfulness, and illuminating the path to a life imbued with balance and serenity.

1. The Breath as a Source of Renewal

At the heart of harmonious living lies the understanding of breath as a perpetual source of renewal. This section explores how conscious breathwork serves as a continual process of rejuvenation—cleansing the mind, invigorating the body, and replenishing the spirit. The breath, like a gentle river, becomes the elixir that sustains and revitalizes every facet of our being.

2. Mindful Breathing in Relationships

Breathwork extends its transformative touch into the realm of relationships. This subsection illuminates the practice of mindful breathing as a foundation for harmonious connections. By bringing conscious breath awareness into interactions, individuals navigate relationships with patience, empathy, and presence, fostering an atmosphere of understanding and compassion.

3. Breath as a Guide in Decision-Making

In the complexities of decision-making, the breath emerges as a steady guide. This section explores how conscious breathwork becomes a contemplative practice—a moment of pause before decisions are made. By attuning to the breath, individuals access a space of clarity and intuition, making choices that resonate with their deepest wisdom and values.

4. Cultivating Gratitude through Breath

Gratitude becomes an art woven into the breath. This subsection delves into how breathwork becomes a vessel for cultivating gratitude. Through intentional breaths that acknowledge the present moment and the gift of life, individuals foster an attitude of gratitude that permeates their daily experiences, inviting joy and appreciation.

5. Breath and Emotional Resilience

Emotional resilience blossoms through the rhythmic dance of breath. This section explores how conscious breath practices become allies in navigating the ebb and flow of emotions. By embracing emotions with breath awareness, individuals develop resilience, allowing them to respond to life's challenges with grace, equanimity, and a centered heart.

6. Breathwork for Stress Management

In the face of stress, breathwork emerges as a potent tool for management. This subsection delves into specific breath techniques tailored for stress relief. Whether through calming breaths that activate the relaxation response or energizing breaths that invigorate the body, practitioners harness the power of breath to navigate stress and cultivate inner balance.

7. Breath as a Bridge to Mindful Presence

Mindful presence unfolds as the breath becomes a bridge to the present moment. This section explores how conscious breathing anchors individuals in the here and now. By infusing breath awareness into routine activities, from walking to eating, individuals cultivate mindfulness, savoring the richness of each moment and fostering a deep connection with life.

8. The Breath as a Teacher of Patience

Patience, a virtue often tested in the tapestry of life, finds its teacher in the breath. This subsection illuminates how breathwork becomes a practice of patience. Through rhythmic and intentional breaths, individuals learn to embrace the unfolding of each moment with patience, allowing life to reveal its lessons at its own pace.

9. Integration of Breath in Self-Care Rituals

Self-care becomes a sacred ritual with the integration of breathwork. This section guides individuals to weave conscious breathing into their self-care practices. From breath-awareness meditation to breath-infused relaxation techniques, individuals create a sanctuary of well-being, nurturing the body, mind, and spirit through the gentle embrace of breath.

In Chapter 7, breathwork transforms from a practice into a way of living—a harmonious dance with life's rhythms. May this exploration inspire practitioners to infuse every breath with mindfulness, fostering a life where breath becomes the gentle conductor orchestrating a symphony of balance, serenity, and well-being.

7.1 Nurturing Relationships through Breath

In the intricate dance of human connections, the breath emerges as a subtle yet profound catalyst for fostering harmony and understanding. This section explores the art of nurturing relationships through conscious breathwork, unveiling the transformative power of the breath in creating bonds enriched with presence, empathy, and shared moments of mindfulness.

1. The Breath as a Bonding Force

At the core of nurturing relationships is recognizing the breath as a shared and unifying force. This subsection illuminates how conscious breathing becomes a communal experience, weaving a tapestry of connection between individuals. By synchronizing breath in shared moments, whether through intentional pauses or harmonious breath patterns, relationships deepen, transcending words to communicate on a deeper, soulful level.

2. Mindful Breathing in Communication

Communication thrives when infused with the mindfulness of breath. This section explores the practice of mindful breathing during conversations. By bringing conscious awareness to the breath while listening and speaking, individuals foster genuine presence. This mindful exchange nurtures understanding, allowing each participant to feel heard and valued in the sacred space of shared breath.

3. Breath as a Tool for Empathy

Empathy, the cornerstone of meaningful connections, finds expression through breath. This subsection delves into how conscious breathwork becomes a tool for cultivating empathy. By attuning to the breath, individuals tap into the emotional currents of others, creating a space where understanding and compassion flow effortlessly. Breath becomes the bridge that connects hearts in moments of joy, sorrow and shared humanity.

4. Breathwork for Conflict Resolution

In the face of conflict, breathwork emerges as a gentle mediator. This section explores specific breath techniques that support conflict resolution. Individuals navigate turbulent emotions by engaging in calming breaths, fostering a state of emotional equilibrium. In shared breathwork, conflicting parties may find a bridge to understanding, transforming discord into an opportunity for reconciliation.

5. Cultivating Presence in Shared Activities

Shared activities become enriched through the cultivation of breath awareness. This subsection illuminates how engaging in activities— whether cooking, walking, or creating together—can be infused with conscious breath. As individuals synchronize their breath with the rhythm of shared endeavors, they create a harmonious flow that enhances connection and deepens the joy of shared experiences.

6. Rituals of Breath Connection

Integrating breath connection into relationship rituals becomes a sacred practice. This section explores the creation of rituals that involve intentional breathing. Whether through shared breath-awareness moments before parting ways or synchronized breaths as a daily greeting, individuals establish rituals that infuse relationships with a sense of reverence, fostering a bond that transcends the ordinary.

7. Breath as a Source of Patience and Understanding

Patience and understanding flourish in the garden of conscious breath. This subsection delves into how intentional breathing becomes a source of patience during challenging moments in relationships. By taking a pause, connecting with the breath, and allowing a moment of stillness, individuals create a space for understanding to blossom, diffusing tension and nurturing the seeds of harmony.

8. Reflection and Gratitude in Relationship Breathwork

Breathwork becomes a canvas for reflection and gratitude within relationships. This section guides individuals to engage in breathwork practices that involve reflection on shared experiences and expressions of gratitude. By infusing breath with reflection and thankfulness, relationships become an ongoing journey of mutual growth and appreciation.

In relationships, breathwork becomes a silent maestro orchestrating the symphony of connection. May this exploration inspire practitioners to infuse their relationships with the mindfulness of breath, creating a harmonious dance where each breath becomes a note in the melody of shared understanding and love.

7.2 Cultivating a Harmonious Life

Harmony is an art woven into the fabric of daily living, and breath emerges as a guiding brushstroke in this masterpiece. In this section, we delve into the practice of cultivating a harmonious life through conscious breathwork—an art that transforms the mundane into the sacred, fostering balance, mindfulness, and a deep connection with the rhythms of existence.

1. The Breath as the Rhythm of Life

At the heart of a harmonious life lies the understanding that breath is the rhythm of existence itself. This subsection illuminates how conscious breathwork aligns individuals with the universal cadence, creating a symphony where each breath resonates in harmony with the ebb and flow of life. By recognizing the breath as the sacred pulse, individuals attune themselves to the inherent balance within and around them.

2. Mindful Breath in Daily Rituals

Daily rituals become an avenue for cultivating mindfulness through breath. This section explores how ordinary activities, from morning routines to meals, can be elevated into sacred rituals through conscious breathwork. By infusing each action with mindful breathing, individuals create a harmonious tapestry where even the simplest gestures become acts of presence and reverence.

3. Breath as an Anchor in Chaos

Amid life's chaos, the breath becomes an unwavering anchor. This subsection delves into the practice of using conscious breath as a stabilizing force during challenging moments. By turning to intentional breaths in times of stress or uncertainty, individuals cultivate resilience, fostering a sense of calm that allows them to navigate the storms of life with grace.

4. Breathwork for Emotional Equilibrium

Emotional equilibrium unfolds through the art of breathwork. This section explores how conscious breathing becomes a palette for balancing emotions. By engaging in breath practices that harmonize the breath with emotional states, individuals create a canvas where emotions are acknowledged, embraced, and transformed into a harmonious expression of inner balance.

5. Breath as a Path to Mindful Decision-Making

Mindful decision-making unfolds as individuals attune to the breath. This subsection illuminates how conscious breath becomes a guide in the decision-making process. By taking intentional breaths before making choices, individuals create a space for clarity and discernment, allowing decisions to emerge from a place of inner wisdom and alignment with their values.

6. Breath and Gratitude in Daily Reflection

Daily reflection becomes infused with the gratitude of breath. This section guides individuals in incorporating breathwork into reflective practices. By taking moments of intentional breathing during daily reflection, individuals cultivate gratitude for the experiences, lessons, and connections life offers, creating a harmonious dance with the ever-unfolding narrative of their journey.

7. Breath Connection in Nature

Connecting with nature becomes a harmonious communion through breath. This subsection explores how conscious breathwork unfolds in outdoor experiences. Whether walking in nature, practicing breath awareness under the open sky, or breathing in the scent of flowers, individuals harmonize with natural rhythms, fostering a deep sense of interconnectedness with the earth and all living beings.

8. Integration of Breath in Sleep Rituals

The realm of sleep becomes a sanctuary for breath and renewal. This section guides individuals in integrating breath practices into sleep rituals. By engaging in calming breaths before bedtime or incorporating breath awareness during moments of wakefulness in the night, individuals create a harmonious transition into the realm of dreams, allowing the breath to guide them into restful slumber.

In the canvas of everyday life, conscious breathwork becomes the brushstroke that paints a harmonious masterpiece. May this exploration inspire practitioners to infuse each moment with the mindfulness of breath, creating a life where harmony unfolds as a natural expression of their connection with the sacred dance of existence.

Chapter 8: Advanced Pranayama Techniques

As the journey of Pranayama deepens, Chapter 8 unveils a realm of advanced techniques that beckons practitioners to explore the subtle dimensions of breath mastery. These techniques, rooted in ancient wisdom and refined through the ages, offer a profound gateway to heightened states of awareness, spiritual insight, and a harmonious union with the breath's transcendent potential.

1. The Art of Kevala Kumbhaka

At the pinnacle of breath control, Kevala Kumbhaka stands as a jewel—a state where breath retention occurs effortlessly and spontaneously. This section delves into the intricacies of Kevala Kumbhaka, guiding practitioners to cultivate a state where the breath naturally dissolves into stillness. By surrendering to the innate wisdom of the breath, individuals open a portal to profound states of meditation and heightened spiritual awareness.

2. Nadi Shuddhi: Purifying the Energy Channels

Nadi Shuddhi, or alternate nostril breathing, transcends its foundational form to become a gateway for purifying the subtle energy channels. This subsection explores advanced variations and nuances of Nadi Shuddhi, guiding practitioners to balance and purify the nadis (energy channels) with precision. Through intricate breath patterns, individuals harmonize the flow of prana, unlocking deeper dimensions of vitality and spiritual awakening.

3. Surya Bhedana and Chandra Bhedana

The solar and lunar aspects of breath, Surya Bhedana, and Chandra Bhedana offer advanced techniques to channel solar and lunar energies within the body. This section delves into the practices of selectively activating either the right or left nostril to access specific qualities of energy. By aligning breath with the cosmic energies, practitioners harmonize with the rhythms of nature, awakening dormant potentials and balancing polarities.

4. Brahmari Pranayama: The Humming Bee Breath

Brahmari Pranayama transcends its gentle hum into an advanced technique for vibrational healing and spiritual elevation. This subsection explores variations of Brahmari, incorporating specific pitches and durations. Practitioners learn to harness the transformative power of sound vibration within the body, awakening higher states of consciousness and attuning to the cosmic resonance.

5. Ujjayi Pranayama: Whispering Ocean Breath

Ujjayi, the oceanic breath, evolves into an advanced practice that deepens the connection between breath and inner sound. This section guides individuals to refine Ujjayi, emphasizing the subtle sound produced within the throat. By immersing in the rhythmic whispering of the oceanic breath, practitioners access a state of tranquil awareness, transcending the boundaries of the physical body.

6. Shitali and Sitkari: Cooling Breath Variations

Shitali and Sitkari, the cooling breaths, extend into advanced variations that unlock the body's potential to regulate temperature and balance internal heat. This subsection explores techniques for extending the duration and intensity of Shitali and Sitkari, facilitating a profound cooling effect on the nervous system. Practitioners harness these breaths to cultivate inner coolness and enhance mental clarity.

7. Agni Sara: Fire Essence Technique

Agni Sara, the fire essence technique, becomes an advanced practice that stokes the inner fire of digestion and transforms it into a potent force for spiritual awakening. This section guides practitioners to master the intricacies of Agni Sara, incorporating advanced variations to refine abdominal locks and channel prana into the core. Through this mastery, individuals awaken the dormant spiritual fire within.

8. Antar Kumbhaka: Inner Breath Retention

Antar Kumbhaka, or inner breath retention, unveils an advanced dimension of breath mastery that transcends external control. This subsection explores practices that guide practitioners to retain the breath within, redirecting the focus from external breath control to internal absorption. By diving into the ocean of inner stillness, individuals access heightened states of meditation and self-realization.

In Chapter 8, practitioners embark on an advanced exploration of Pranayama, where breath transcends its ordinary nature to become a sacred vehicle for spiritual awakening. May this chapter inspire a dedicated and mindful journey into the profound depths of breath mastery and the limitless possibilities it holds for the sincere seeker.

8.1 Progressive Breath Mastery

In the pursuit of advanced Pranayama, the journey of breath mastery becomes a progressive exploration, unfolding layers of subtlety and refinement. This section illuminates the path of progressive breath mastery, guiding practitioners through stages of refinement and deepening awareness to attain the pinnacle of Kevala Kumbhaka—the spontaneous and effortless state of breath retention.

1. Cultivating Breath Awareness

The foundation of progressive breath mastery rests upon cultivating an unwavering awareness of the breath. This subsection introduces practices that refine the art of observing the breath—its texture, rhythm, and nuances. By developing acute sensitivity to the breath's ebb and flow, practitioners lay the groundwork for a journey of profound exploration.

2. Balancing Inhalation and Exhalation

The harmonious dance of inhalation and exhalation is a key element in progressive breath mastery. This section explores techniques for balancing the duration and intensity of inhalation and exhalation. Through conscious adjustments, practitioners refine the symmetry of the breath, fostering equilibrium in the subtle energies flowing within the body.

3. Seamless Transitions Between Breaths

Progressive breath mastery involves seamlessly transitioning between different breath phases. This subsection guides practitioners in cultivating fluidity between inhalation, exhalation, and moments of retention. By eliminating abruptness in transitions, individuals create a continuous and rhythmic flow, deepening their connection with the breath's inherent grace.

4. Extending the Duration of Breath Phases

Advancing in breath mastery entails extending the duration of each breath phase deliberately. This section introduces techniques for gradually lengthening inhalation, exhalation, and breath retention. Through patient exploration, practitioners expand their lung capacity and refine their ability to sustain breath phases, paving the way for advanced practices.

5. Incorporating Mudras and Bandhas

Mudras and Bandhas, subtle energy locks, become integral in progressive breath mastery. This subsection explores how specific hand gestures (mudras) and energetic locks (bandhas) can be incorporated to enhance breath control. By engaging these subtle tools, practitioners refine their ability to direct and channel prana, deepening the transformative potential of their breathwork.

6. Internalizing Kevala Kumbhaka

Kevala Kumbhaka, the pinnacle of breath mastery, unfolds as practitioners internalize the state of spontaneous breath retention. This section guides individuals in letting go of conscious control, allowing the breath to enter a state of effortless stillness. Through patience and surrender, practitioners access the profound realm where breath retention occurs spontaneously, revealing the limitless dimensions of meditative awareness.

7. Integrating Breath Mastery into Meditation

As breathe mastery progresses, it seamlessly integrates into the practice of meditation. This subsection explores how advanced Pranayama becomes a gateway to meditative states. By merging breath control with focused attention, practitioners transcend the ordinary boundaries of thought, entering realms of heightened awareness and inner stillness.

8. The Art of Sustained Samadhi

In the culmination of progressive breath mastery, individuals touch the realms of sustained Samadhi—a state of profound meditative absorption. This section delves into practices where breath becomes a vehicle for entering and sustaining Samadhi. Practitioners navigate the subtle currents of breath to dissolve into the ocean of pure consciousness, experiencing the unity of self with the infinite.

In the progressive journey of breath mastery, practitioners unfold the layers of their being, diving into the depths of awareness and transcending the limitations of the breath. May this exploration inspire a dedicated and mindful progression, leading individuals toward the sublime states of Kevala Kumbhaka and the transformative realms of meditative consciousness.

8.2 Breathwork for Transformation

Within the realm of advanced Pranayama, breath becomes an alchemical force, capable of catalyzing profound transformation on physical, mental, and spiritual levels. In this section, we delve into breathwork practices designed for transformative experiences, guiding practitioners to harness the breath as a potent tool for inner metamorphosis.

1. Purification through Kapalabhati

Kapalabhati, the breath of fire, takes on a transformative role in cleansing and purifying the body. This subsection explores advanced variations of Kapalabhati, intensifying the rapid breath cycles to amplify the cleansing effect. Practitioners engage in this transformative breathwork to release toxins, invigorate the nervous system, and create a purified vessel for spiritual exploration.

2. Pranic Energization with Bhastrika

Bhastrika Pranayama, the bellows breath, unfolds as a dynamic practice for pranic energization. This section guides practitioners in advanced Bhastrika variations, elevating the intensity of breath cycles. Through this transformative breathwork, individuals draw upon prana—the vital life force—infusing the body with renewed energy and awakening dormant potentials for heightened awareness.

3. Nauli Kriya: Manipulating Internal Energy

Nauli Kriya, a yogic cleansing technique, becomes a transformative practice for manipulating internal energy. This subsection introduces advanced Nauli variations, guiding practitioners in isolating and moving the abdominal muscles. By channeling breath and energy into specific regions, individuals stimulate digestive fire, enhance organ function, and unlock the transformative potential within the body.

4. Anulom Vilom: Balancing Dualities

Anulom Vilom, or alternate nostril breathing, transcends its balancing qualities to become a tool for resolving dualities within the mind. This section explores advanced Anulom Vilom techniques, incorporating extended breath ratios. Practitioners engage in this transformative breathwork to harmonize the dualistic aspects of the mind, fostering mental clarity and a deep sense of inner equilibrium.

5. Bastrika Kumbhaka: Breath Retention in Bellows Breath

Bastrika Kumbhaka, the breath retention phase within Bhastrika, emerges as an advanced practice for internal stillness. This subsection guides individuals in extending the duration of breath retention during Bhastrika, creating a transformative pause that amplifies the meditative aspect of the practice. Through this breathwork, practitioners access profound states of inner calm and heightened awareness.

6. Integrating Sound in Ujjayi Pranayama

Ujjayi Pranayama transforms with the integration of sound as a catalyst for transformation. This section explores advanced Ujjayi variations, emphasizing the audible quality of the breath. By consciously creating a rhythmic sound within the throat, practitioners enhance the transformative potential of Ujjayi, facilitating a deeper connection with the inner self.

7. Sankalpa and Breath Manifestation

Sankalpa, the power of intention, aligns with breath to become a transformative force. This subsection introduces practices where individuals set clear intentions during specific breath phases. By combining breath awareness with focused intention, practitioners harness the transformative energy of the breath to manifest positive changes in their lives.

8. Pranayama in the Silence of Antar Mouna

Antar Mouna, inner silence, becomes a transformative space where breathwork leads to profound stillness. This section guides individuals to engage in breathwork as a preparation for entering the meditative state of Antar Mouna. Through intentional breath practices, practitioners create an inner sanctuary of silence, allowing transformative insights and self-realization to emerge.

In the crucible of advanced Pranayama, breathwork becomes a transformative journey, unraveling the layers of the self and awakening latent potentials. May this exploration inspire practitioners to engage in breath practices that catalyze profound transformation, leading them towards the sublime realms of self-discovery and spiritual awakening.

Conclusion:

In the tapestry of existence, the breath emerges as a thread that weaves through the realms of mind, body, and spirit, creating a harmonious symphony of life. As we conclude our journey through "The Art of Pranayama," we stand at the threshold of a profound understanding—the transformative power of conscious breathwork to cultivate a life of balance, vitality, and spiritual awakening.

A Journey Inward: Rediscovering the Breath

Our exploration began with the recognition that the breath is not merely a physiological process but a sacred bridge connecting us to the essence of our being. From the foundational practices of breath awareness to the intricate techniques of advanced Pranayama, we embarked on a journey inward—a journey where each inhalation and exhalation became a step towards self-discovery.

Mind-Body Connection: The Breath as the Nexus

Throughout these pages, we delved into the intricate dance between mind and body, understanding how the breath serves as the nexus that unites these realms. Breath awareness became a gateway to mental clarity, emotional resilience, and physical well-being. Through the art of breath control, we harnessed the innate intelligence of the breath to harmonize the intricate facets of our being.

Spiritual Odyssey: Breath as a Path to the Divine

In the chapters exploring spirituality and Pranayama, we uncovered the sacred dimension of breath—a conduit to the divine within and around us. From deepening spiritual practices to exploring advanced techniques that transcend the ordinary, we touched upon the transformative potential of the breath to elevate consciousness and lead us to states of oneness and transcendence.

A Harmonious Life: Breath as the Conductor

Our journey culminated in the understanding that the art of Pranayama is, at its essence, a journey towards a harmonious life. The breath, when consciously harnessed, becomes the gentle conductor orchestrating a symphony of balance, serenity, and well-being. It guides us in relationships, decision-making, and daily rituals, infusing each moment with mindfulness and a deep connection to the rhythm of existence.

Empowerment through Breath Mastery

As practitioners of the art of Pranayama, we stand empowered with the tools to master the breath—a key to unlocking the potential within. Whether embracing foundational practices or venturing into the realm of advanced breath mastery, we have witnessed the transformative capabilities of conscious breathing to catalyze change, foster resilience, and awaken the dormant energies that reside within us.

The Unending Journey: Breath as a Lifelong Companion

Our exploration of Pranayama is not a destination but a lifelong journey—an ever-unfolding odyssey of self-discovery and growth. The breath, our faithful companion, remains a teacher, guide, and source of renewal throughout our lives. As we continue to refine our breath practices, may the journey be a constant reminder of the infinite possibilities that unfold when we harmonize with the rhythm of our breath.

In concluding "The Art of Pranayama," let us carry forward the wisdom gained, the practices embraced, and the transformative potential of each mindful breath. May the art of Pranayama continue to be a source of inspiration, guiding us towards a life that resonates with balance, vitality, and the harmonious dance of mind, body, and spirit.